Intermittent Fasting:

Beginner's Guide to Intermittent Fasting for Effective Weight Loss

Greg Austin

DEDICATION

This book is dedicated to my beautiful wife and children. You drive and inspire me to be a better man each and every day.

CONTENTS

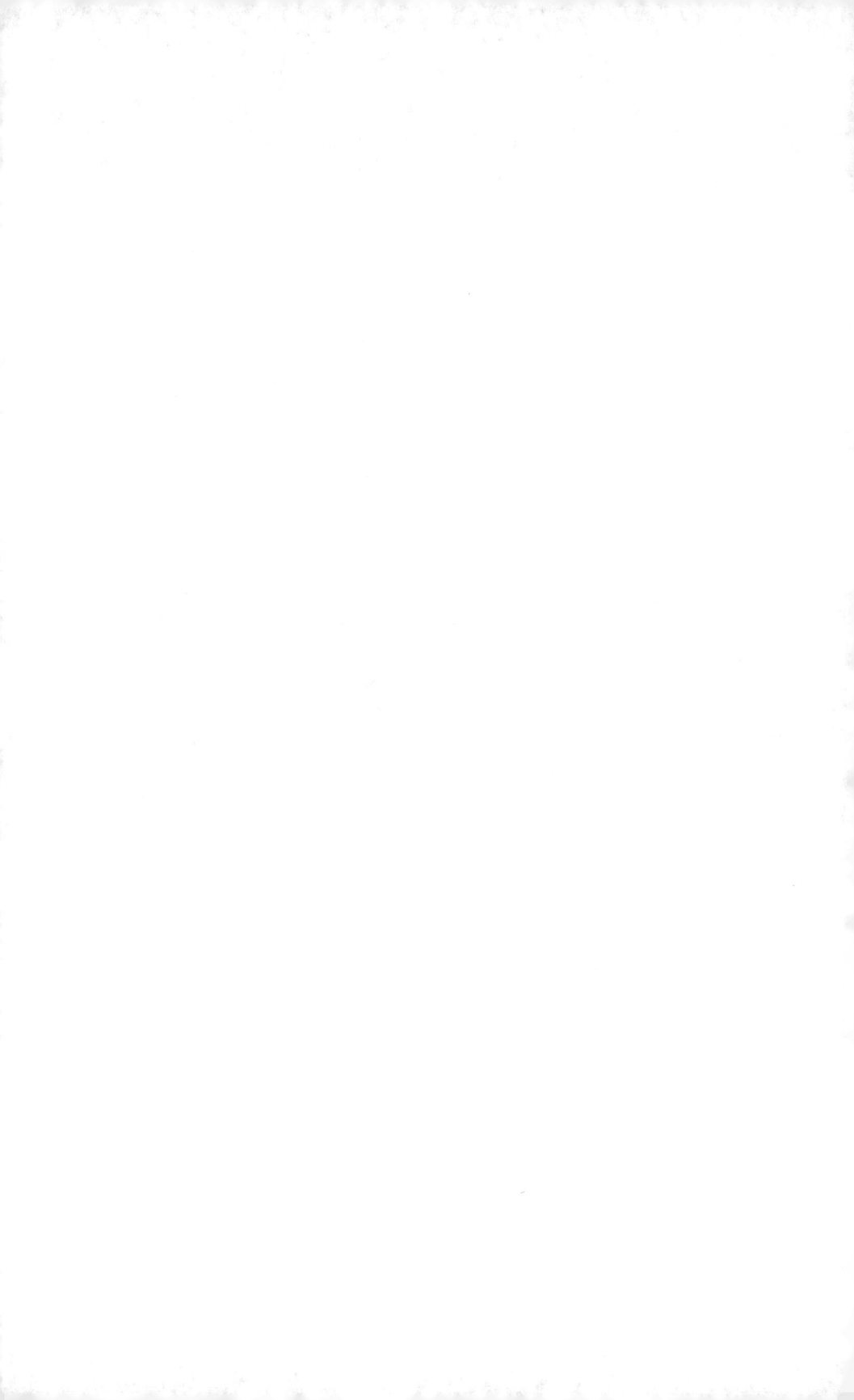

INTRODUCTION

Haven't we always been told that breakfast is the single most important meal of every day? That if we eat nothing else, we shouldn't skip that one? And how many different rules have you heard about losing weight? "You must eat a good breakfast to get your metabolism going", or "breakfast like a king, lunch like a prince and dinner like a pauper". Or what about, "you must eat 5 or 6 small meals a day to keep your metabolism operating properly".

All of these rules seem to be so ingrained now that they are accepted as gospel but I'm here to tell you that you have my permission to ignore them. Completely and utterly. There is absolutely no truth in any of these so-called rules and there is also no proof that eating breakfast is the only way to lose weight and feel healthier.

So, what can help you to lose weight? Well, I want to tell you about a new way of eating, a way of eating that has been proven to work, scientifically and in practice. This way of eating promotes skipping meals for the most optimum body fat burning process, the maximum amount of muscle retention and for a more efficient body.

I want to talk to you about intermittent fasting, about how it works and how you will feel so much healthier, fitter and more energetic, as well as dropping the pounds that just won't shift any other way. Intermittent fasting is a highly controversial subject because it turns everything we have ever been taught completely on its head but, by the end of my book I hope that you can see exactly how it works and that all of the myths that you have heard over time are just that – simply myths.

CHAPTER 1: WHAT IS INTERMITTENT FASTING?

intermittent fasting is NOT, is another diet so don't look at it that way. In fact, intermittent fasting, although it takes a while to get into it, will become a way of life to you. To start with it will involve you having to make very conscious decisions not to eat every meal, to skip certain ones – which ones depends on which style of intermittent fasting you choose to follow but I will talk more about those in a later chapter.

Fasting and then eating on purpose means that your caloric requirements are all eaten during a specific window of time and you choose not to eat any food outside of those times. There are several ways to do intermittent fasting for it to work properly and for the best benefit:

- Eat regularly during a set period of time. For example, only eat between the hours of 12 noon and 8 PM which mean, horror of horror, you don't eat breakfast. Some people opt for a 6-hour window while other take it even further and only eat during a 4-hour window of time.

- On one day, skip out two meals, which mean you go 24 hours without eating anything at all. For example, if you eat on your normal daily schedule and have your last meal at 8 PM, you don't eat anything else until 8 PM the following day.

OK, so you are most likely thinking, if you skip a meal, you are eating less, therefore you will lose weight more quickly. Well, that is only partly true. By skipping a meal, you can eat more on your other meal and still consume fewer calories but, as anyone who has been on a diet knows, one calorie is not the same as another one. Not only that, the timing of your meals plays an important part.

How Does It Work?

When you start intermittent fasting, you have two phases – "fast" and "feast" – and your body will work differently on each one. When you have eaten, your body goes into processing mode, taking a few hours to sort out your food. It burns off what it can and because this is a steady source of fuel, one that is readily available, your body is going to use that as energy rather than the fat stored in your body. This is even truer if your meal consisted of sugar and carbohydrates as the human body looks for sugar as its first form of energy.

When you fast, your body doesn't have the luxury of a ready source of fuel so it has to turn to the fat stores in your body for energy instead of glucose or glycogen. And we all know that, when our fat stores are used, we lose weight. This also works when you go to the gym or exercise while fasting. Because your body doesn't have a supply of glycogen or glucose to fuel itself, it will turn to the fat stores in the body and burn it as energy.

So why does this work? Because, when we eat, our bodies react to the energy we flood it with by producing insulin. The more sensitive you are to the insulin, the more likely it is that you will use up the energy from the food more efficiently, thus creating muscle mass and losing weight. The human body is highly sensitive to insulin following a fasten period so it makes sense that fasting is the way to go

The energy that is not used or stored as fat is stored in the liver and muscles as a starch called glycogen. When you sleep or fast, this glycogen is depleted and, when you work out, it is depleted even more. This leads to even more insulin sensitivity and this means that, when you eat after training or after a fast, the energy is stored much more efficiently – this is mostly going to be as glycogen, burned up as an energy source and a very tiny amount stored as fat.

Now compare all of this to a normal day, when you eat normally and you don't fast intermittently. Your insulin sensitivity is at a normal level and the food you eat will quickly fill your glycogen stores, leave enough glucose in your blood to be used as energy and the rest will be stored as fat.

When you fast, your body produces more of the Human Growth Hormone (HGH) (the same thing happens when you sleep) and, when you combine this with a lower production of insulin, which leads to more insulin sensitivity, your body is being primed for faster muscle growth and faster fat loss.

To put this in simple terms, intermittent fasting helps to teach your body to make better and more efficient use of the food you eat. So why does everything you read tell you to eat several smaller meals throughout the day? There are several reasons why:

1. When you eat, more calories are used to burn/process the food so, in theory, if you eat 6 small meals a day, your body is burning calories on an almost constant basis and your metabolism is firing on all cylinders. Sorry, but that doesn't work. It really doesn't matter if you sit and eat 2000 calories in a 6-hour window or spread across the entire day, you are still eating 2000 calories and your body will burn off the same number in processing the food. So next time someone tells you that you should eat little and often you can tell them that it is a load of rubbish and doesn't work.

2. Eating smaller meals means that you won't overeat when you eat your main meal of the day. There may be some truth in this, especially if you find portion control hard or have no idea what you should be eating. However, once you teach yourself how to eat properly, eating 6 times in one day can seriously cramp your style and it means expending a lot of effort. And, because of the smaller meals, you are never likely to feel full and will be more likely to eat more with the next meal or snack.

OK, so this small and often principle may seem logical but point number one above shows why it won't work unless you struggle with portion control. Think – go back in time to the caveman. Do you seriously think that they ate 6 times a day on schedule? No, they ate when they could and their bodies were fully adapted to working properly during times when they couldn't eat.

The most important thing to remember is, it isn't how much you eat, it is what you eat. If you eat the right foods, you definitely do not need to eat so frequently and you will find intermittent fasting a great deal easier.

CHAPTER 2: THE UPS AND DOWNS OF INTERMITTENT FASTING

As with every diet and with every way of eating or life, there are the usual pros and cons. Nothing works for everyone but, as there are several different styles of intermittent fasting, don't give up if one doesn't work for you; just have a short break and then try another plan. Let's look at the ups and downs of intermittent fasting:

Pros

- **You can lose fat fast -** most of the studies that have been carried out on how intermittent fasting affects the rate of fat loss also look at how calories are restricted a well. One study on obese women showed that if they combined a restriction in calories with liquid meals, they lost more body fat and showed a vast improvement in their cardiovascular health, reducing the risk of heart disease quite significantly. With intermittent fasting, because you are restricting your food intake to a specific window of time, it follows that you should, in theory, take in fewer calories.

- **Your digestive system gets a break** – on a normal diet, with the three or six meals a day plus the snacks in between, your digestive system is never given a break and can become compromised. This can lead to all sorts of conditions such as leaky gut syndrome, which means your intestines have become "leaky" with tiny holes allowing for substances that are not normally allowed through to sneak into your bloodstream causing problems. Intermittent fasting gives your digestive system a break from the work and gives it time to recover and to repair itself.

- **Your fat stores will be reduced** – when you go long periods without eating, your body will start to use up your fat stores. When you eat, your insulin levels rise and you could end up storing fat. So, when you snack between meals, your insulin production is raised more and more fat is stored. However, if you restrict your food intake to a specific window, as you do in intermittent fasting, your insulin levels are raised less and your fat cells are given encouragement to let go of some of the fat for energy.

- **You see food in a different light** – As a nation, we tend to eat pretty much constantly and we quickly lose sight of the value of food. When you do intermittent fasting, you get to stand back a little and take stock of the relationship you have with food. You can examine why you gravitate toward comfort foods; what emotions cause you to do that. The other problem is that, whether we accept it or not, subconsciously we are scared of going hungry and if you go into intermittent fasting with that feeling you might just be surprised at the mental changes that happen, the clarity with which you start to see things. In other words, intermittent fasting can show you deep into yourself, a few truths that you might just be avoiding, "self-medicating" by eating. To start with, intermittent fasting may be somewhat painful for some of you but once you get over the first hurdle, the long-term benefit will far outweigh the short-term pain.

Cons

- **Can lead to some eating disorders** – Intermittent fasting has something of a "binge and purge" mentality to it and it could, if not followed properly, lead to or make worse cases of bulimia and a number of other eating disorders. Some so-called Intermittent Fasting (IF) experts allow, even push for, an "anything goes" style during the feast stage and that can easily lead to shame and guilt that, over time, will just become worse. However, this is not a common occurrence and will normally only happen where a person already suffers from problems that lead to emotional eating.

- **It may be more harmful to women** – Studies on intermittent fasting show that an alternate day fast/feast program can actually work against women, lowering their tolerance to glucose and could lead to a crash in metabolism. There are also other studies that show intermittent fasting can trigger off a bout of anxiety, sleeplessness, interruption to menstruation, and a dysfunction in the regulation of hormones in women. Stress makes these problems worse so women need to consider all eventualities before they undertake intermittent fasting protocols.

- **It may lead to a food obsession** – intermittent fasting leads to deeper, more meaningful relationships with food but, for some people, this could mean that they end up focusing more on food than ever before. Hunger is a powerful thing and it is the mechanism that kept us alive in early days. These days, food is in such ready abundance for some countries that starvation just isn't going to happen and, as a result, hunger is not something we confront. The problem comes when you think you are starving; everything else falls to the wayside and food becomes the main focus and, with intermittent fasting, that could lead to obsession.

- **It could lead to a reliance on coffee** – most of the intermittent fasting plans include coffee because caffeine is a stimulant that can help you to keep going when you don't eat. If you are a coffee drinker and you are on an intermittent fasting plan, you might find that you end up drinking more coffee than is actually good for you. Caffeine will make already high cortisol levels worse and that makes it more difficult to burn off fat and you run the risk of muscle breaking down.

- **It could lead to an increase in food intolerances** – while you might break your fast with a nice healthy meal of lean chicken and broccoli, the tendency is there to reward yourself with something unhealthy. Hunger tends to take control of any discipline or logic and, while some experts do advocate that you eat what you want during the feast period, it can lead to intolerances, spikes in blood sugar, followed by severe crashes, cravings, inflammation and lot of other problems

Obviously, the cons might just put some people off doing intermittent fasting but, as with anything, provided you do it properly, the benefits are there. If you are looking for a quick weight loss fix, then IF is not the diet strategy for you. It is a long term health strategy and when done incorrectly can cause harm to the body. When participating in intermittent fasting, make sure you know exactly what you are doing and follow an appropriate plan that is outline by experts.

That said, if you do just want a quick fix, need to get into that outfit in a hurry, you can try intermittent fasting but keep these suggestions in mind:

- Keep the caffeine to a minimum. Just one cup a day and then stick to green tea, which contains theanine for calming and EGCG for fat burning.

- Make sure your meals are planned well ahead of time. This will stop you from obsessing about food or overeating when you break your fast.

- You may be hungry when you break the fast but you must not take in huge amounts of food – not only will it not make you feel good; it will undo all the benefits of your fast.

- Help keep your cortisol levels down by taking up yoga, meditation or deep breathing.

- Take BCAA's – branched-chain amino acids – every couple of hours when fasting to curb cravings and appetite as well as lowering levels of cortisol

Intermittent Fasting Without Feeling Hungry

What if you are looking to have a go at intermittent fasting but don't want to fast for long periods of time? Try one of these two ways:

- Skip the main dinner twice a week. Eat a decent breakfast and lunch and then you will go a pretty impressive 18-20 hours before you eat again. Use the above tips to stop yourself from getting hungry.

- The second way is even easier if you really don't want to skip a meal. A study carried out on mice found that, when they were only able to eat during an 8-hour window, they lost a lot more fat and were much healthier than those or who ate whenever they wanted, even though both groups of mice were on exactly the same food. In the same way, you can gain the benefits from intermittent fasting by restricting your eating window to 12 to 14 hours per day. Eat a healthy and good-sized meal at around 6 PM and then eat nothing else until 8 AM, when you should consume a breakfast rich in protein. This will give you a fasting window of 13 hours approximately and, with any luck, you will be asleep for a good part of those.

That means there will be little to none of the feelings of deprivation or hunger that comes with longer fasts but you still get the benefits.

CHAPTER 3: THE MOST POPULAR INTERMITTENT FASTING PROGRAMS

Every day we hear of another fad diet hitting the streets. No fat, high fat, high carb, low carb, little and often, gluten free, etc., etc. All of these so-called diets are apparently proven to help you lose weight quickly but they do not always work for every person.

The real secret to losing weight, feeling healthier and improving your body composition lies in skipping a meal here and there, going for several hours with little to no calorie consumption. For some people, this can be very easy and the benefits are well worth it. When you think about it logically, every single one of us fasts for several hours every day – while we sleep. All you do when you start an intermittent fasting plan is extend those hours and being more conscious about what you eat and when.

But, is this the right way for you and which intermittent fasting plan is the best one for you? The following are the top five intermittent fasting plans, all tested and tried. Before we look at those, let's go back to the 1930's. As far back as then, scientists have been looking into the effect of cutting meals to cut calories. One scientist from the USA found that, by cutting calories significantly, mice in one study lived for much longer and were healthier. In recent times, studies have noted the same thing in monkeys, roundworms and fruit flies, showing that a cut of 30 to 40% in calories, however it is done, can result in a third more life span. There is also significant data to show that, by limiting the amount of food we eat, we also limit the risk factors of several common illnesses and diseases. There are also those who believe that fasting can increase the response to insulin, thus helping to cut down on cravings and hunger.

The top five intermittent fasting plans are about taking full advantage of these benefits. Each of these plans are designed for different groups of people giving them better results over one of the other intermittent fasting plans. Never force yourself to follow a method that is not suited to you because it simply won't work. So chose a plan that is the best matched to you.

The first step to starting on intermittent fasting is to read through the following plans. Each one will tell you how long you should fast for and give you guidelines on what to eat, as well as telling you the type of person it is aimed at. Remember one thing – intermittent fasting is not for everyone and if you suffer from a health condition you should only undertake IF with the explicit consent of your doctor.

Leangains

This plan is best suited to the dedicated gym rat who wants to build up their muscle and lose body fat.

How Does It Work?

Women should fast for 14 hours, 16 for men every day. That gives you a feeding window of 8 to 10 hours. During the fasting, no calories should be consumed, although you may drink black coffee, use sweeteners that are free of calories, drink diet soda and eat sugar-free gum. It also won't hurt if you add a small splash of milk to your coffee. Most people who do this one find it easiest to have the bulk of their fasting period overnight while they sleep and breaking their fast about 6 hours after getting up the next day. This can be adapted to your own schedule but you must have a constant window for feeding otherwise your hormones will become unregulated and you will struggle to stick to it.

The food you consume during that feeding window will depend on when you are working out. When you exercise, you should eat more carbohydrates than fat and, on days where you don't exercise, a higher intake of fat is more important. Protein needs to be high every day although there are various factors that will affect your intake – your goals, age, gender, activity levels, and body fat. Most of your food should be made up of unprocessed whole foods but, if you really do not have time for a proper meal, you can eat a meal replacement bar or drink a protein shake.

Pros

For a lot of people, the biggest benefit is that you don't have to stick to a meal plan, you can pretty much eat when you want within your feeding window. Most people do find it easier to stick to three meals as this is how we are programmed.

Cons

While there is a good deal of flexibility in when you eat during your window, there are some pretty tight guidelines on what you should eat. You must work out which days you are working out on and tailor your food to high carb, low fat and the opposite on days when you don't work out. Because the nutrition plan is a bit strict and you must schedule your meals around your workouts, it can be tough for some people to stick to.

Warrior Diet

This one is best for those who are sticklers for the rules.

How Does It Work?

The Warrior diet requires you to fast for around 20 hours every day, eating just one large meal in a four-hour window at night. However, you can't just eat anything because a key part of this one is in when you eat and what you eat. The philosophy revolves around giving your body the nutrients that it requires while remaining synchronized with your circadian rhythm – the fact that humans are evolved as nocturnal feeders and are programmed to eat at night also helps here.

Rather than actually going 20 hours without any food at all, the fasting period so more about eating less. You may consume a few portions of raw vegetables or fruit, drink fresh organic juice and eat a little protein if you want. The effect of this is to maximize your body's fight or flight response, which in turn promotes energy, alertness and stimulates body fat burning.

Your four-hour window for eating is at night, in order to maximize the body's ability to recuperate and relax, promoting a sense of calm and helping the digestive system while also giving your body the required nutrients to do that.

Night eating can also help the body in its production of hormones and in day-time fat burning. What you eat is important as is the order that you consume the food groups– start off with a meal of fat, protein and vegetables. If you are still hungry when you finish that, then you can add on carbohydrates.

Pros

This works for some people because you can still eat small amounts during the fasting period, thus increasing energy and fat burning

Cons

Although it is nice to be able to eat something rather than going hungry the food and nutrition guidelines are very strict and you could find that it has an impact on your social life. On top of that, eating just one main meal at night might not be easy for some, especially if you are not a fan of eating large amounts late in the day

Alternate Day Diet

This one is designed for those who are disciplined with a specific goal in mind in terms of weight loss.

How Does It Work?

This one is actually quite easy to follow. You simply eat normally one day and eat only small amounts the next day. On those days, your calorie intake should be around one-fifth of your normal intake. So, if your normal intake is 2000 calories, your alternate day should only be 400 calories. To make these days easier to bear, it is recommended that you opt for protein shakes in place of meals because they tend to contain the nutrients you need. They can also be sipped at throughout the day instead of consumed in one sitting as a meal. However, you should really only use these for a maximum of 2 weeks and then you must start to eat proper food. If you are a regular gymgoer, you might want to schedule your workout days for when you eat normally rather than a low-calorie day.

Pros

This is all about losing that weight so, if this is your goal, consider this method carefully. On average, those who cut down their calorie intake by around 20 to 35% can expect a weight loss of up to 2.5 lbs. every week.

Cons

While this is quite an easy one to follow, bear in mind that you might find it tempting to binge on a normal day. Stay on track by making sure your meals are planned out fully ahead of the day so you are not caught heading for a fast food place or one of those eat all you can buffets while you are starving hungry.

Feast/Fast

This one suits the gym lovers who long for a cheat day

How Does It Work?

If you can't find anything in the plans talked about above, this one may be for you. It takes the best out of those three methods and puts it all together in one nice plan. You get a cheat day every single week that is followed by a fast for 36 hours and then the rest of the week is split up between the different protocols. It might be best to work this one so that your fast day falls on a busy day when you need to focus your attention on something other than eating

Pros

While, technically, we all fast every day, most of us do it in a somewhat disorganized way and that is why we can't reap the benefits. This plan offers a full weekly schedule so that your body gets used to it and you get to enjoy a full-on cheat day.

Cons

If you can't handle a cheat day by eating properly and only indulging in your favorites in moderation, then this might not be the right method for you. You need to be able to stop eating when you are full and not overdo it on the unhealthy treats. Also, this is quite a specific plan and, because the fasting period differs each day, it might be a little difficult for those who like a set schedule in their routine every day.

Eat Stop Eat

This one is suited to those who eat a healthy diet but just want a bit of a boost.

How Does It Work?

Moderation is the key to this one. You can eat pretty much what you want but just not as much as you would normally. If you want a slice of cake, have it, just not the whole cake. You will fast for a period of 24 hours a couple of times each week. During this time, you can consume no food but you can drink as many calorie-free drinks as you want. When the fast period is over you can eat normally. It might be best to start this one after an evening meal so that when the fast is broken it is with your normal meal.

By eating in this way, you will cut your calorie intake over the course of a week without actually limiting yourself too much. You must work out regularly, especially resistance training, if your goals are to lose weight or improve your body composition.

Pros

It might seem like an awfully long time to go without eating but you can be flexible here. You don't have to start out with an all-or-nothing approach. Just go as long as you can without eating to start with and increase that time gradually up to 24 hours. Start on a busy day and where you are not going to be involved in any social obligations that revolve around food.

Another pro to this is that nothing is forbidden, you don't need to count your calories and you don't need to restrict your diet or weigh out your food. Just eat in moderation.

Cons

Some people will find it hard to go 24 hours with no calorie intake, especially to start with. You may suffer from headaches, anxiety, fatigue and bad moods but this will reduce over time. Also, the long period without food can also make it easy to binge when you do eat again. This just takes a little self-control.

Our bodies will always take the time to adjust to a new way of eating and some people will need longer than others. Start slowly and be careful; build up to a full-on fast gradually to give yourself time to get used to it. Just keep in mind that not everyone will benefit from fasting. If you have specific dietary requirements, a medical condition or suffer from a chronic disease, you must consult with your doctor before you start a fast.

If you do intend to give it a go, you must be very self-aware – if the fast is causing you problems or you find that you have to eat something to get you through, there is nothing wrong with that. Stop a fast whenever it makes you feel uncomfortable. It will take time for your body to get used to it as well as your mental attitude. For the women be aware that hormones can get in the way so take it easy. If fasting really doesn't agree with you, stop, try something else.

5 Tips for Your Very First Fast

If you opt to give it a go, keep these 5 tips in mind:

- Make sure you stay hydrated. Drink plenty of water as this will help you to feel fuller as well as help to flush out the toxins in your body.

- Do some of your fast overnight so you are sleeping through it.

- Change the way you think about fasting. See fasting as nothing more than having a break from the daily task of eating, not as if you are being deprived.

- Start on a day when you are tremendously busy and don't have time to think about your next meal.

Get working out. Exercising while you are fasting can give you much better results as well as helping to take your mind off food. You don't have to overdo it but anything is better than nothing.

CHAPTER 4: INTERMITTENT FASTING MYTHS DEBUNKED

Intermittent fasting is nothing new; people spread across the entire globe have been doing it ever since time began, whether by choice or through circumstance. These days, we do it to help control our weight and improve our health but, even with all the evidence and the research that shows the positive benefits, there are still a number of myths that people cling to, myths that are simply not based in reality. Knowing what they are is half the battle to succeeding.

Myth 1 – Fasting burns off your muscle mass

This is probably the most common of all the misconceptions, especially amongst men who are attempting to put on muscle. We often hear that we should be eating several small meals a day to keep the body supplied with calories and energy and it is because of this that many fear fasting will destroy their muscle mass. This is not the case when you intermittent fast. When fasting for short periods of time, your body starts to breakdown glycogen into glucose and it increases the breakdown of fat. It does not start to breakdown muscle fibers.

Now yes, fasting periods of 24 hours or more can have catabolic effects on the body. However, intermittent fasting rarely requires you to fast for that long, usually only up to 18 hours at a time and that does not have any effect on muscle mass. Studies were recently carried out on subjects who fasted every other day for a period of 8 weeks, and the weight loss registered was an average 9 lbs. The real shocker is that all of that weight came from body fat not from muscle mass and, in fact, none of the subjects showed any loss of muscle mass at all.

That said, if you do not follow the fasting plan properly do not eat a healthy diet and do not include exercise, you could run the risk of faster muscle loss and other things that can have catabolic effects are training too hard and too much, cutting your calorie intake drastically in too short a time or doing a lot of cardio exercise. On its own though fasting will not have any negative effects on the preservation of your muscles.

Myth 2 – Fasting slows down metabolism

This is a half-truth rather than a myth because there is some truth to it. When your body is not given nourishment, a survival mechanism automatically kicks in – the lowering of your metabolism. This is a real benefit because, should you ever find yourself in a prolonged period of starvation, it can help you to survive longer.

However, this will only happen if you were to deprive your body of food for days, not hours. Studies show that even in situations where subjects took part in a 72 hour fast, no slow-down in metabolism was noted. And, because intermittent fasting doesn't require you to fast for anywhere near that long your metabolism rate is not going to slow down.

Myth 3 – If you don't eat breakfast you'll get fat

We have had this drilled into us for years – breakfast is the absolute most important meal of the day and if you skip it, you can suffer from weight gain, fatigue, and low concentration levels. However, it has been proved that not eating breakfast will not have any effect on weight gain. Intermittent fasting involves missing the first one or two meals of the day and then starting again with lunch. This is not a bad protocol to follow because it means you are not obligated to have a breakfast just because you've been told it the most important meal. I'm not trying to say that you shouldn't have breakfast, jut that it isn't perhaps as important as it's been made out to be. If you do miss breakfast and get hungry, have a glass of water with a drop of lemon or lime juice in it, to stop the hunger pangs and get a dose of vitamin C.

Myth 4 – Fasting will push your Cortisol levels up

While fasting can certainly push your Cortisol levels up, it is a temporary thing and doesn't happen to everyone. You are more likely to suffer from this if you eat a permanently low-calorie diet.

Myth 5 – Fasting makes your brain foggy

A fact to interest you – 20 % of the nutrients contained in your food are used by your body to regulate your brain function, regardless of the fact that your brain matter actually only takes up 2% of your body. So, logic would dictate that, if you ate less, you would have a harder time concentrating. Science tells a different tale, though. A study that was carried out on the effects of fasting on the brain showed that fasting twice a week can actually have a positive effect on the brain by lowering the decline in cognitive function that is associated with Alzheimer's disease and other forms of dementia.

When you fast, you are actually putting your brain under a small amount of stress. When you exercise, you stress your muscles and they become stronger as a result; the same happens with the brain in that the neurons strengthen up when they are stressed through low energy levels.

Myth 6 – Fasting leads to overeating

Plenty of research has been done on this and it has been revealed that most people who fast only eat a small amount of extra calories on their next meal. One study was carried out on a group of people who fasted for 24 hours and it was showed that, on the next day they only ate an extra 500 calories, a small amount compared to what they would have eaten over the two days.

This requires discipline. You will feel hungry during a fast and the temptation is there to binge eat when you break the fast, as well as eating the wrong food choice. This is seen as some kind of reward for having starved themselves for a period of time. It is important to remember that, when your fast is over, normal service resumes. There's no reward – that will come in the weight loss and the extra energy – and, once you are used to it, you will find that you won't get hungry anyway, at the most it will be nothing more uncomfortable than a bit of a growl in the tummy.

Myth 7 – Exercise will be impacted negatively while fasting

We all know that our bodies need energy and that comes from our food so it would seem to make sense that when you fast, your energy levels are low and you can't exercise as well as normal. So is there any truth to this myth?

Yes, and no, mostly no. Depending on how well you keep yourself hydrated, you should not notice any real impact on your energy levels and performance. That said, we are all different and how much or little we eat and drink affects everybody differently. If you feel like you are drained of energy during a fast, you should perhaps consider using supplements that contain caffeine. Or, you could just refrain from exercising on days when you fast and go back to it when you are eating normally. Eventually, your body will become used to it and you won't notice the effects anyway.

Myth 8 – IF doesn't work for women

There is a certain amount of truth to this as we discussed earlier. Hormones play a big part and women may find it harder to gain the full results out of a fast. However, the results you do gain will not be negative and weight loss will occur if the fast is followed properly.

Myth 9 – IF is independent of a calorie deficit

Those who go on a fast will normally consume a lower amount of calories but that isn't always true. Weight loss is about burning off more calories than you are consuming and if you continue to eat the same amount of calories during a week of fasting that you would on a normal week then wouldn't expect to see any different results than before.

There are a few small benefits to eating little and often but, at the end of the day, 2000 calories are 2000 calories, no matter how and when they are consumed. When you begin a fast, your body will begin to burn off the fat in your body as the energy supply simply isn't there because there are no glycogen stores to turn to. And, as fasting results in higher insulin sensitivity, there is less chance of fat being stored. If you don't maintain the cut in your calorie intake, all the weight you lost will most likely come back.

Myth 10 – Fasting is nothing more than starving

It is not the same as being starved. When you fast, your glycogen levels are depleted and your body starts to burn off body fat for energy. When you are in starvation mode, your fat reserves are completely gone and your body will start to burn muscle tissue. Starvation is fasting at its most extreme. There are those who restrict their food intake severely because they believe it will help them to lose weight. These people are starving, not fasting.

The symptoms tell of yet another difference. When you begin fasting, you might experience mild fatigue, dizziness and a bit of a headache. Once you get into it, these symptoms will disappear. With starvation, the symptoms are far more serious. Muscle wastage, organ failure, cognitive decline, and seizures are not uncommon in people who are starving and if you experience these when you are fasting, you have gone too far. Stop and eat immediately because otherwise the effects may not be reversible. Then go and see your doctor and get some proper help and advice.

CHAPTER 5: FINAL ROUNDUP

By now, you should be well aware of the ins and outs of fasting, of the huge benefits and the possible consequences. You should be aware that, by using intermittent fasting in the correct way for your body, you can lose weight and keep it off and that choosing the right plan is the only way to succeed.

Intermittent fasting is one of the healthiest ways to lose weight and yes, that often means skipping breakfast. Expect your body to go through a good deal of changes as your hormones level out and expect your body to turn into a lean mean fat burning machine – provided you do it right, and I can't stress that enough. Just missing a meal here and there is not considered fasting and you will be more tempted to pig out when you do eat.

There are other benefits to fasting besides weight loss, though. Bigger muscles, prevention of many chronic diseases and even anti-aging can all be considered huge benefits, as well as a general feeling of well-being and higher energy levels. To finish my guide, first, I want to go through my top ten tips for getting started on intermittent fasting, especially if this is your very first time.

1. **Stop eating and start living your life**

Most people are not prepared to give intermittent fasting a go because the concept of going with a meal or two is completely alien to them. Yes, when you are hungry, it does seem daft to consciously deprive yourself of a meal but there is only one reason why you feel hungry – because you are used to eating when you want and your body is used to a regular overload. If you understand that you are in a good place to start with intermittent fasting and you will find it easier to get past the first couple of weeks.

2. **One day at a time**

Really and truthfully, intermittent fasting isn't any different from anything else. If you set out with the intention of doing intermittent fasting forever more, you are going to fall at the first hurdle. The rest of your life is a long time to consider especially as intermittent fasting can extend your life by up to one third. However, if you take it one day at a time, you will find it so much easier to cope with. You will see that you can go 4 to 8 hours without eating and, one the first day is over, the next day will be easier. Keep going, one day at a time, and before you know it, intermittent fasting will be a part of your life.

3. **Know what your goals are**

Preferably before you start. Are you looking to lose weight? If so, how much? Are you looking to improve your body composition? Are you looking to increase your muscle mass? Think about it carefully because your goals will determine the style of intermittent fasting that you do. For example, if you were going for disease prevention and anti-aging, you could get away with a 36 hour fast, whereas for body composition you be looking at a 16 hour fast with an 8-hour window for feeding. Whatever you do, do not fast for more than 72 hours at the very most.

4. Set up your intermittent fasting around your social life

Yes, you can actually fast all day and have your feeding window in the evening but consider this – it has been proven that, by doing this kind of fast, you will eat more in terms of calories and you are more likely to cheat – all the time. Take your social obligations into account when you set your intermittent fasting hours and try not to have it so you are eating very late at night.

5. Drink water in the morning

Most people find that it is easier to set their fasting so that the main part of it is done overnight, while they sleep. This means you have just a few waking hours to go without food so, to overcome those initial hunger pangs first thing in the morning, drink a glass of water the minute you wake up. While you sleep, your body dehydrates and we all know that dehydration gives off signals that are similar to hunger. Water first thing in the morning will replenish some of what you lost and will also eliminate much of the hungry feeling you have.

6. Make it easy on yourself – drink tea and coffee

If you are fasting through the morning, drink some tea – just don't add any milk or sugar to it. Just drink it straight and warm and it will do a few things – eliminate hunger pangs and help you to focus better. If you are not a tea drinker, have a cup of coffee, again, no sugar or milk/cream. Some people drink a bulletproof coffee that is made from coffee, butter, and MCT oil or coconut oil. You might think that this is going to be extremely high in calories and you would be right. But these calories are different because your body will burn them off straight away as energy without getting in the way of things like cell repair. Give it a go and see how you get on with it

7. **Remember that you are not going to be hungry forever more**

When you feel hungry it is because your hormones are kicking off, having a bit of a hissy fit. The only reason for this is because they have become used to being fed on a regular basis – sometimes too regular. You get hungry in the morning because your body is used to you eating then. Give it a few weeks on intermittent fasting and you will find that those hunger pangs disappear as your body get used to your new regime you will be mentally prepared and will now that you won't be hungry; psychologically you will be much healthier and your body will follow.

8. **Choose your cheat day and eat wisely**

Some people like to have a cheat day when they are fasting, a day when they can eat whatever they like. Instead of pigging out on everything that is bad for you, keep it in moderation. Foods like almond butter, extra dark chocolate, and sweet potatoes are healthy choices and much cleaner than milk chocolate, muffins and chips. Don't undo all of your hard work with one day of indulgence – or over-indulgence.

9. **Keep busy while you fast**

This is why most people opt to fast overnight because they are asleep and not thinking about food. If your fast spills into waking hours, keep busy. Go for a walk, catch up on all the work you have been putting off, do anything that takes your focus away from food, especially when you are just starting out on a fast for the first time.

10. **Your food choices really do matter**

While you might find that intermittent fasting is a fantastic way to prove your health and overall weight, it really won't make any different if you don't eat the right foods while in the feast stage of the fast. Try to eat a diet that is low in carbohydrate and high in fat and protein unless you are on a workout day, in which case, you need to eat less fat and better carbohydrates

11. **Intermittent fasting is not for everyone**

Make no mistake; intermittent fasting is not going to suit all of us. Try and monitor exactly how you feel before determining if it is right or not. While it is a very healthy practice it will not work for all and, if it doesn't work for you, don't persevere with it. Just give it up to experience and move on to something else. There are also people who should not do intermittent fasting but I will talk a bit more about those later on.

10 Reasons Why Skipping Breakfast Is Good for You

OK, so, throughout this guide, I have talked on several occasions about missing out that most important of all the meals in a day – breakfast. To expound on that theory, I want to tell you just 10 of the best reasons why you should miss breakfast out of your day, why having a meal at that time of day is what makes you feel constantly hungry and stops you from losing weight. So, why miss breakfast:

1. **To burn off fat**

You already know that the act of fasting allows body fat to be released and burnt off as fuel. The reason I because of extra low levels of insulin which, as we also know, is released when we eat. So, a short period of fasting turns your body into a fat burning machine. When you fast overnight, do not eat breakfast when you get up. Leave it a few hours, go do some exercise and drink some water. The benefits will soon show for themselves.

2. **To stop chronic hunger**

Fasting has the effect of suppressing hunger and going without breakfast is far easier than eating it and then trying to stop yourself once you have started. Breakfast is, in effect, nothing more than the mechanism to open the floodgates to binging. Eating breakfast can result in you gaining weight and it can make you incredibly irritable simply because all you are doing is counting time until you can eat again. Fasting is a fantastic way to cut down on anxiety related to food and eating and, because you will be eating within a set window of time, you will feel much fuller for longer because all your calories will be eaten in that window.

3. **To stop the aging process**

Nobody wants to look old before their time but, unfortunately, the stresses of life take their toll on us, as does being out in the sun and not drinking enough water. Intermittent fasting works by giving your body the chance to get rid of damaged cells, a process that is vital to stopping you from looking old and maintaining your youthful looks for longer.

4. **To help the immune system**

Studies have shown that fasting for 48 hours can help your body to fight diseases. This works because, when you fast, your body triggers off the process of regenerating white blood cells and this has major implications for people who have a damaged or compromised immune system, such as those with cancer or other diseases.

5. **To cut down on chronic inflammation**

Low-grade inflammation in the body is associated with high body fat levels. This is not good news because it is associated strongly with hypertension, rheumatoid arthritis, fatty liver asthma, atherosclerosis, diabetes cardiovascular disease, insulin resistance, cancer, and aging. Not a nice list of diseases; a list that can be conquered by following an intermittent fasting plan properly.

6. **To help prolong your life**

Intermittent fasting is an excellent way to drop the weight and to help keep it off. The advantages of this are not just in a more stable weight, you also get to lower your risk factors for heart disease, heart attacks, strokes, high cholesterol, cancer, diabetes and high blood pressure all of which are potential killers lying in wait.

7. **To increase your longevity**

Not only does fasting help you to lose weight, it can also increase your productivity quite significantly. Because you won't be eating, you will have more time for work, for relationships and to spend time with your family.

8. **To increase your focus**

Fasting boosts the Sympathetic Nervous System, which is the dominant system and is in control of your fight or flight instincts. Because this is sharpened while you are fasting, your focus and concentration are also much sharper

9. **To improve mood**

Fasting causes higher and more concentrated levels of BDNF– brain-derived neurotrophic factor and this has a positive effect on your mood.

10. **So you can consume carbs at night**

If you fast all day, you eat at night and this is natural because human beings are inherently programmed to eat at night. So, by skipping breakfast and lunch you can happily eat carbs at night and not worry about piling on the pounds.

Is Fasting Safe for Me?

Most people will find that intermittent fasting, no matter what format they follow, is a fantastic way of losing weight and improving their overall heath. However, unfortunately, there are some people who simply cannot do intermittent fasting for one reason or another. Fasting as an effect on hormones, particularly those growth hormones and that means certain groups of people cannot fast because it would not be healthy for them.

Intermittent fasting should not be carried out by:

- Children
- Teenagers who have not stopped growing
- Women who are expecting a baby
- Women who are breast-feeding a baby
- Anyone who has just undergone surgery
- Anyone who suffers from an eating disorder
- Anyone who has insulin-controlled diabetes
- Anyone who is underweight

There are also certain medications that are not a particularly good fit with intermittent fasting and if you are taking any of these, you need to check with your doctor before you start any fasting protocol:

- If you are currently taking warfarin

- If you suffer from any medical condition that has resulted in a weak immune system
- If you are taking any form of medication that has to be taken with food

If you do not fall into any of these categories and are doing intermittent fasting, there are times when you may want to consider stopping:

- If you feel at all unwell
- If you feel ok but are definitely running a fever
- If you are suffering from a high level of stress

If you are ever in any doubt whatsoever, you should always stop what you are doing and consult your doctor immediately. Continuing with a fasting protocol when you shouldn't be can be dangerous to your health.

What Happens When You Fast for Too Long?

Fasting is an incredibly powerful way of improving your health and losing weight but there are ways of doing it that are not considered to be healthy. If for example, your fast involve little to no calorie intake for a period of 5 days or more, you run the risk of something called "refeeding syndrome". This usually happens within 4 days of you beginning to eat again and it can cause some serious side effects – lung trouble, heart problems, muscle problems – and, if it isn't caught early enough, it can be fatal. It is for this reason that there are set protocols for intermittent fasting and most will never advocate you going for more than 36 hours without any calories or 3 days when you are on a low-calorie intake

Always follows the guidelines properly to ensure maximum benefits and good health while fasting.

If you are unable to start intermittent fasting for one reason or another, there are other ways that you can help yourself to keep in shape and lose the weight. You can cut sugar and bad carbohydrates from your diet, stick to whole and unprocessed foods, eat organic and drink plenty of water. Learn about nutrition, about what your body needs to operate efficiently and what it most definitely doesn't need Exercise on a regular basis and stay active. Above all, be consistent in your approach.

CONCLUSION

I want to thank you for taking the time to read my guide on intermittent fasting. I truly hope that you now understand how beneficial fasting is to you, how it can help you to lose weight where all those other diets have failed miserably. Intermittent fasting, done properly, is absolutely the best way to get in shape.

Despite the fact that there is nowhere near as much research on the subject, mostly down to a lack of money, there is sufficient evidence to prove that intermittent fasting really does work for most people. I can't say for everyone because, as you clearly saw in my last chapter, there are some people that simply cannot do intermittent fasting for one reason or another. I will say that it is very dangerous to undertake a fasting protocol if you are not physically fit enough to do it, or if you can potentially cause harm to your body by doing it.

Fasting requires more than just not eating for a few hours. It requires incredible willpower; it requires a certain amount of strength, both physical and mental and if you don't possess any of that then you will fail in your bid. There are a number of protocols that you can follow but it is absolutely vital that you are honest with yourself when you are choosing which way to go. Each plan is set for a specific type of person and following the wrong one will ensure failure because you will not be able to follow it without losing heart.

Lastly, before you start any intermittent fasting protocol, make sure you know exactly what is expected for it to succeed. Educate yourself about nutrition, about what your body needs to work, the different minerals and vitamins. Then learn which foods contain them and make sure that when you are on the feast period of your fast that you eat a properly balanced diet.

Sugar, candy, pastries, and muffins may have been major food groups to you before but, when you are fasting they are not even a part of your life, except in tiny amounts so be prepared not to binge on them when you can eat.

Once again, thank you for reading my guide and I wish you lots of luck in your intermittent fasting journey.

ABOUT THE AUTHOR

Greg Austin is an outgoing fitness lover, with a passion for helping people grow more whole, both physically and mentally. Along with enjoying indoor fitness, such as weight lifting and resistance training, he also enjoys outdoor activities such as hiking, whitewater rafting, snowboarding, and playing football. He is a dad, a husband, and a friend who is always striving to create a healthy life for him and his family.

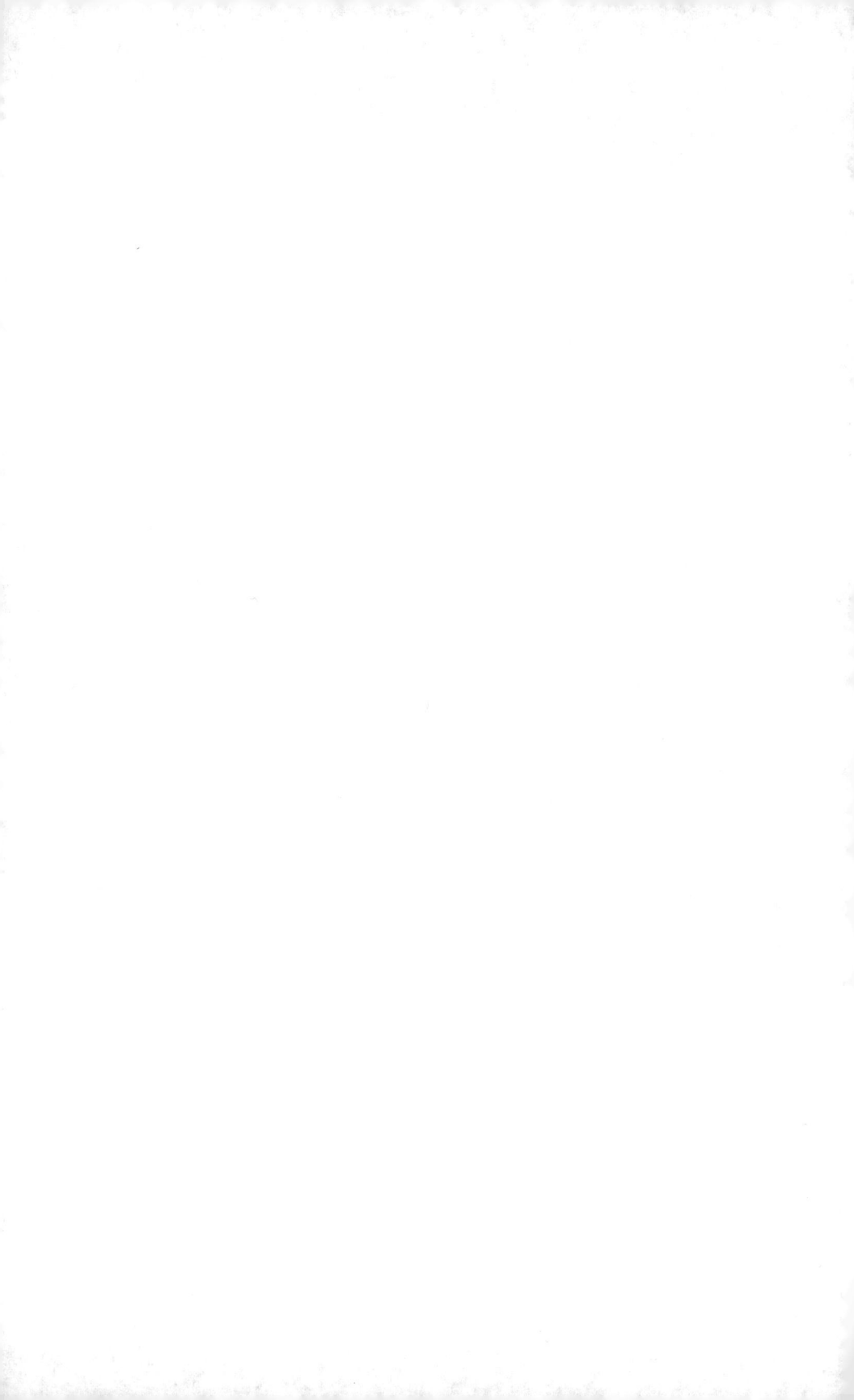

www.ingramcontent.com/pod-product-compliance
Lightning Source LLC
Chambersburg PA
CBHW060650290526
45793CB00001B/483